ANTI-INFLAMMATORY DIET

FOR NOVICES

Enriched Recipes, Foods, Meal Plan &
Procedures To Approach And Resolve
Gut Inflammation, Lupus, Arthritis
And Other Health Crises

DR. MATEO GABRIEL

DISCLAIMER

The information in this book is only meant to be used for general reading. In any way, the author and publisher do not promise or represent that the information in this work is full, correct, reliable, appropriate, or available. This includes any warranties that are expressed or implied. Because of this, you should only rely on this material at your own risk.

This book is not meant to replace professional help. If you have any questions about a subject, you should always get help from a qualified expert. The author and distributor of this book are not responsible for how the information in it is used or abused.

The author's thoughts and feelings are shown in this book. They do not necessarily represent the official policy or stance of any other person, group, employer, or business.

Any third-party material that you can get to through this book is not endorsed or backed by the author or publisher.

The information in this book is correct at the time it was published, after all possible checks. However, the author and distributor are not responsible for any loss, damage, or inconvenience that may be caused by mistakes or omissions.

TABLE OF CONTENTS

CHAPTER ONE 10

INTRODUCTION TO ANTI-INFLAMMATORY DIET 10

KNOWING ABOUT INFLAMMATION 10

MEANING AND CATEGORIES.............................12

THE BODY'S ROLE IN INFLAMMATION 14

CHAPTER TWO 16

THE CONNECTION BETWEEN HEALTH AND
INFLAMMATION..16

DISEASE AND CHRONIC INFLAMMATION 16

INFLUENCE ON TOTAL WELL-BEING....................17

THE SCIENCE OF INFLAMMATION........................18

MOLECULAR AND CELLULAR MECHANISMS 20

MEDIATORS INFLAMMATORY.............................21

CHAPTER THREE 24

LOW DIET IN INFLAMMATION 24

AN ANTI-INFLAMMATORY DIET'S FUNDAMENTALS
....24

COMPARING PROCESSED AND WHOLE FOODS 25

THE VALUE OF MAKING NUTRIENT-DENSE...........26

CHAPTER FOUR 30

ESSENTIAL ANTI-INFLAMMATORY DIETS 30

FRUITS AND VEGETABLES 30

FOODS HIGH IN OMEGA-3 FATTY ACIDS 31

HERBS AND SPICES...32

CHAPTER FIVE 34

RECIPES FOR MEAL PLANNING AND AVOIDED FOODS
....34

INFLAMMATORY CATALYSTS 34

COMMON SENSITIVITIES AND ALLERGENS 35

EXAMPLES OF MENUS...36

COOKING ADVICE FOR A LIFESTYLE LOW IN 38

CHAPTER SIX 40

LIFESTYLE TECHNIQUES...40

EXERCISE AND PHYSICAL ACTIVITY 40

FUNCTION IN INFLAMMATION REDUCTION 41

CHOOSING THE BEST EXERCISE FOR YOU 42

STRESS MANAGEMENT 43

KNOWING THE RELATIONSHIP BETWEEN STRESS
AND INFLAMMATION 44

RELAXATION TECHNIQUES....................................45

OPTIMIZING YOUR SLEEP......................................45

IMPORTANCE OF HIGH-QUALITY SLEEP 46

ADVICE FOR DEVELOPING BETTER SLEEP HABITS .47

CHAPTER SEVEN 48

SUPPLEMENTS AND PROTOCOLS FOR REDUCING
INFLAMMATION..48

A SYNOPSIS OF SUPPLEMENTS 48

CRUCIAL MINERALS FOR INFLAMMATION............49

POSSIBLE DANGERS AND ADVANTAGES 50

HERBAL TREATMENTS..50

CONVENTIONAL AND RESEARCH-BASED 51

INCLUDING HERBS IN YOUR DAILY ROUTINE 52

PROTOCOLS FOR REDUCING INFLAMMATION......53

COLLABORATING WITH MEDICAL EXPERTS 54

CHAPTER EIGHT 56

MONITORING DEVELOPMENT AND MODIFYING THE
PROCEDURE 56

KEEPING AN EYE ON INFLAMMATION LEVELS 56

SCREENS AND BIOMARKERS 57

IDENTIFYING IMPROVEMENTS..............................58

MODIFYING YOUR PROCEDURE 61

KEEPING YOUR BODY IN MIND 63

LOOKING FOR EXPERT ADVICE.............................64

CHAPTER ONE

INTRODUCTION TO ANTI-INFLAMMATORY DIET

KNOWING ABOUT INFLAMMATION

An intricate biological reaction, inflammation is essential to the body's defense systems and the healing process. The immune system, blood arteries, and other signaling molecules are all involved in this meticulously controlled and highly coordinated sequence of events. This reaction is necessary to preserve tissue homeostasis and protect the body from any dangers. It can be brought on by several stimuli, including infections, damaged cells, or irritants.

Inflammation, in its broadest sense, is the body's defense mechanism against damaging stimuli. This dynamic process entails a sequence of actions intended to remove the insult that caused the necrotic cells and tissues, as well as the inflammatory cells that ensued. Acute and chronic inflammations are the two primary forms of inflammation. Acute inflammation is an instantaneous, swift reaction that usually lasts a short while, whereas chronic inflammation lasts longer and is frequently linked to several illnesses.

MEANING AND CATEGORIES

Classic symptoms of acute inflammation include redness, swelling, heat, discomfort, and loss of function. The body is attempting to heal and restore normal tissue function, as seen by these symptoms. The process is highly regulated and involves a series of actions coordinated by blood vessels, immune cells, and signaling molecules like chemokines and cytokines. Acute inflammation's main objectives are to remove the source of cell damage, remove damaged cells, and start the healing process of injured tissue.

Conversely, chronic inflammation is a more protracted and persistent reaction that can aid in the emergence of several illnesses, such as cancer, neurological diseases, and autoimmune disorders. In contrast to acute inflammation, chronic inflammation is defined by a persistent activation of the immune system that causes tissue damage and persistent dysfunction. This kind of inflammation is distinguished by the simultaneous influx of immune cells, tissue destruction, and attempts at healing.

THE BODY'S ROLE IN INFLAMMATION

The body uses inflammation for a variety of purposes. Apart from its defensive role against injury and infection, inflammation plays a vital role in the immune system's monitoring and defense processes. It is essential for the elimination of harmed or infected cells, the attracting of immune cells to the site of damage, and the initiating of many molecular pathways that synchronize the response as a whole.

Moreover, inflammation contributes to tissue homeostasis under normal physiological circumstances and is not limited to external dangers such as infections or injuries. The body has sophisticated feedback mechanisms to control inflammation, preventing very strong or persistent reactions that could be harmful. Disturbances in the control of inflammation can give rise to many ailments, underscoring the intricate equilibrium necessary for the appropriate operation of the immune system and general well-being.

CHAPTER TWO

THE CONNECTION BETWEEN HEALTH AND INFLAMMATION

DISEASE AND CHRONIC INFLAMMATION

A protracted and dysregulated immune response known as chronic inflammation has been identified as a critical component in the onset and course of many illnesses. Chronic inflammation can last for a long time, in contrast to acute inflammation, which is the body's normal, transient reaction to an injury or infection. Numerous medical illnesses, including diabetes, neurological diseases, cardiovascular diseases, and several forms of cancer, have been related to the emergence of this persistent inflammatory state. The inflammatory process can cause harm to organs and tissues, which aids in the etiology of some illnesses. It is essential to comprehend the complex relationship between chronic inflammation and disease to create preventive and treatment plans that work.

INFLUENCE ON TOTAL WELL-BEING

Chronic inflammation affects general health in addition to the way certain diseases present. Empirical evidence indicates that an extended period of low-grade inflammation could be linked to various symptoms such as depression, exhaustion, and cognitive impairment. Because inflammation is systemic, it can impact different organs and systems across the body, which can lead to a reduction in general health and vigor. Furthermore, chronic inflammation has been linked to the aging process; some experts suggest that chronic inflammation contributes to age-related diseases as well as the general reduction in physiological function that comes with aging.

THE SCIENCE OF INFLAMMATION

The immune system uses the intricate biological reaction known as inflammation to shield the body from dangerous stimuli including infections, damaged cells, and irritants. A series of actions are involved in the process, beginning with the release of signaling molecules upon danger identification. Consequently, immune cells are drawn to the site of injury and begin to eradicate the threat while facilitating tissue regeneration. Although acute inflammation plays a vital role in defense, chronic inflammation results from an imbalance in the regulatory mechanisms that govern this response. Numerous variables, including genetic predisposition, environmental effects, and lifestyle choices, can lead to dysregulation.

MOLECULAR AND CELLULAR MECHANISMS

At the cellular level, many immune cells, including neutrophils, lymphocytes, and macrophages, work in concert to cause inflammation. These cells release a variety of signaling chemicals that control inflammation, including chemokines and cytokines. A major function of molecular pathways like the nuclear factor-kappa B (NF-κB) pathway is to control the expression of genes linked to inflammation. Although the cellular and molecular mechanisms that underlie inflammation are strictly regulated, an imbalance in these mechanisms can result in chronic illnesses and chronic inflammation.

MEDIATORS INFLAMMATORY

A complicated web of signaling molecules, including prostaglandins, cytokines, and reactive oxygen species, mediates inflammation. By transferring messages between cells and adjusting the immune response, these mediators function as messengers. Tumor necrosis factor-alpha (TNF-α) and interleukin-6 (IL-6) are examples of pro-inflammatory cytokines that are important in enhancing the inflammatory cascade.

Conversely, anti-inflammatory cytokines, such as interleukin-10 (IL-10), support tissue healing and assist in reducing inflammation. Immune homeostasis depends on the careful balancing act between pro- and anti-inflammatory mediators. A disruption in this equilibrium may result in persistent inflammation and play a role in the development of numerous illnesses.

There is a complex relationship between inflammation and health that involves interactions across cellular, molecular, and systemic processes. In addition to acting as a common factor in the emergence of numerous illnesses, chronic inflammation has a profound impact on general health.

Developing focused therapies to lessen the negative effects of chronic inflammation on health requires an understanding of the science underlying inflammation, the cellular and molecular mechanisms involved, and the function of inflammatory mediators.

CHAPTER THREE

LOW DIET IN INFLAMMATION

AN ANTI-INFLAMMATORY DIET'S FUNDAMENTALS

The foundation of an anti-inflammatory diet is the reduction of inflammation in the body and the promotion of general health. It emphasizes consuming foods that have been demonstrated to have anti-inflammatory qualities, which may reduce the risk of chronic illnesses and enhance overall health. The emphasis on real foods over processed ones is one of the diet's main tenets. The body's natural anti-inflammatory activities are aided by the vital nutrients and antioxidants found in whole meals, which include fruits, vegetables, lean meats, and whole grains.

COMPARING PROCESSED AND WHOLE FOODS

Processed foods, as opposed to whole meals, can contain unhealthy fats, preservatives, and additives that can aggravate inflammation. Selecting whole foods is in line with the notion that the body can control inflammation and preserve equilibrium when it is fed a diet high in organic, unprocessed foods. People who adopt an anti-inflammatory diet try to lower the risk factors for inflammation and promote long-term health by consuming fewer processed foods.

THE VALUE OF MAKING NUTRIENT-DENSE DECISIONS

Choosing foods that are high in nutrients is another essential component of an anti-inflammatory diet. In comparison to their calorie level, foods that are high in nutrients have a high concentration of vitamins, minerals, and other vital nutrients. Nutrient-dense foods include fruits, vegetables, nuts, seeds, and seafood, which not only provide a variety of vitamins and minerals but also include bioactive substances with anti-inflammatory qualities. These substances, which include omega-3 fatty acids and polyphenols, are essential for controlling the body's inflammatory response.

The focus on nutrient density in an anti-inflammatory diet also includes encouraging a balance of macronutrients, such as healthy fats. Walnuts, flaxseeds, and fatty fish are good sources of omega-3 fatty acids, which have been related to anti-inflammatory properties. On the other hand, when taken in excess, an imbalance of omega-6 fatty acids—which are frequently present in processed oils and some grains—may lead to inflammation. Maintaining an anti-inflammatory diet requires careful attention to the ratio of omega-3 to omega-6 fatty acids

Choosing whole, unprocessed foods and nutrient-dense options are the cornerstones of an anti-inflammatory diet, as they support the body's natural anti-inflammatory processes. Let's sum up. By concentrating on these ideas, people may be able to decrease inflammation, minimize the chance of developing chronic illnesses, and improve their general health.

CHAPTER FOUR

ESSENTIAL ANTI-INFLAMMATORY DIETS

FRUITS AND VEGETABLES

Including a range of fruits and vegetables in your diet is essential for reducing inflammation. These plant-based diets are high in fiber, antioxidants, vitamins, and minerals—all of which help to lower inflammation in the body. High levels of antioxidants found in berries like raspberries, strawberries, and blueberries can help fight inflammation and oxidative stress. Leafy greens, such as kale and spinach, are rich in phytochemicals and vital elements that have anti-inflammatory and general health-promoting qualities. Furthermore, vitamin-rich colored veggies like tomatoes and bell peppers add to a well-rounded, anti-inflammatory diet.

FOODS HIGH IN OMEGA-3 FATTY ACIDS

Omega-3 fatty acids are essential for reducing inflammation and promoting general health. A great source of omega-3s, specifically EPA (eicosapentaenoic acid) and DHA (docosahexaenoic acid) are fatty fish, such as salmon, mackerel, and sardines. It is well known that the body produces less inflammatory chemicals when these fatty acids are present. Plant-based sources of alpha-linolenic acid

(ALA), a kind of omega-3 fatty acid, include walnuts, chia seeds, and flaxseeds. Maintaining a healthy omega-3 to omega-6 ratio in the diet is important for controlling inflammation. Eating these foods can assist.

HERBS AND SPICES

For millennia, people have utilized herbs and spices for their therapeutic qualities as well as to improve the flavor of food. Numerous spices and plants have bioactive ingredients with anti-inflammatory properties. For instance, curcumin, a strong anti-inflammatory and antioxidant ingredient, is found in turmeric. Another spice with anti-inflammatory and immune-boosting properties is ginger. Garlic, with its sulfur-containing components, has been examined for its potential to alleviate inflammation. Including a range of herbs such as rosemary, thyme, and oregano in cooking can contribute to the overall anti-inflammatory effects of a well-rounded diet.

Adopting an anti-inflammatory diet means embracing a varied range of foods that can help treat inflammation at the cellular level. Fruits and vegetables supply critical minerals and antioxidants, while omega-3-rich diets contribute to a healthy balance of fatty acids.

CHAPTER FIVE

RECIPES FOR MEAL PLANNING AND AVOIDED FOODS

INFLAMMATORY CATALYSTS

Anyone looking to adopt an anti-inflammatory lifestyle must have a thorough understanding of the causes that cause inflammation. Although the body naturally responds to injury or illness with inflammation, persistent inflammation can result in several health problems. Certain foods worsen inflammation by acting as triggers. Foods that have been heavily processed and are high in harmful fats and refined carbohydrates can cause inflammation to rise. Moreover, consuming large amounts of processed and red meats has been associated with elevated levels of inflammatory markers. Identifying and comprehending these triggers is the first step towards controlling inflammation with food decisions.

COMMON SENSITIVITIES AND ALLERGENS

Although each person has a different set of allergies and sensitivities, some foods are generally more likely to cause negative reactions than others. Wheat and other grains include gluten, which is a common allergy for some people and can cause diseases like celiac disease. Some people may have sensitivity to dairy products, especially milk and cheese, which can lead to inflammation and discomfort in their digestive tracts. Understanding one's sensitivities and allergies is crucial because they can have a big impact on inflammation. Elimination diets may help people recognize and stay away from these triggers, enabling them to customize their food patterns to meet their requirements.

EXAMPLES OF MENUS

Creating anti-inflammatory and well-balanced meal planning is essential to controlling inflammation and advancing general health. A colorful assortment of fruits and vegetables, high in antioxidants that reduce inflammation, might be included in a sample meal plan. Fatty fish, such as salmon, are high in omega-3 fatty acids, which are also important in lowering inflammation. Brown rice and quinoa are two examples of whole grains that make great substitutes for processed grains. Lean proteins such as chicken, beans, and lentils provide the meal plan with more nutritional content. Spices and herbs with anti-inflammatory qualities, such as ginger and turmeric, can add flavor.

COOKING ADVICE FOR A LIFESTYLE LOW IN INFLAMMATION

A key component of keeping an anti-inflammatory lifestyle is cooking. Choosing to cook food using techniques like grilling, steaming, or baking as opposed to frying helps keep food's nutritional value intact. An anti-inflammatory diet is aided by favoring healthy oils over saturated fats, such as avocado or olive oil. Experimenting with herbs and spices can provide possible anti-inflammatory benefits in addition to improving flavor. Making meals ahead of time can assist in ensuring that nutrient-dense and anti-inflammatory items are always on hand. Furthermore, drinking enough water and herbal teas to stay hydrated promotes general health and helps to lower inflammation.

As a result, leading an anti-inflammatory lifestyle entails recognizing and avoiding inflammatory triggers, figuring out common allergies and sensitivities, planning well-balanced meals, and using cooking techniques that give anti-inflammatory components priority. People can take proactive measures to manage inflammation and promote long-term health and well-being by adopting these ideas into their daily lives.

CHAPTER SIX

LIFESTYLE TECHNIQUES

EXERCISE AND PHYSICAL ACTIVITY

Maintaining general well-being requires regular exercise and physical activity. Numerous health benefits, such as lowered risk of chronic diseases, improved cardiovascular health, and improved mental well-being, have been associated with frequent physical activity. Fitting exercise into your schedule is crucial for encouraging an active and healthy lifestyle when it comes to lifestyle recommendations. Finding an exercise regimen that works for you and your tastes, whether it be strength training, flexibility exercises, or cardiovascular activities like cycling or running, is essential to creating a long-lasting fitness regimen.

FUNCTION IN INFLAMMATION REDUCTION

Regular exercise has a major, albeit little-known, benefit in lowering inflammation levels in the body. Numerous health problems, such as diabetes, autoimmune illnesses, and cardiovascular disease, are linked to chronic inflammation. It has been demonstrated that exercise modifies the inflammatory response and fosters an anti-inflammatory milieu within the body.

It is believed that one of the ways that exercise promotes general health and prevents disease is through its anti-inflammatory effects.

CHOOSING THE BEST EXERCISE FOR YOU

Choosing the best kind of exercise is a subjective and unique choice. It entails taking into account elements including fitness objectives, inclinations, and any current medical issues. The secret is to discover activities that you enjoy and can regularly include in your schedule, whether they are mind-body practices like yoga and Pilates, strength training with weights, or cardiovascular workouts like walking or swimming. This improves your physical health and fosters a positive outlook, which increases the likelihood that you will continue your exercise routine over time.

STRESS MANAGEMENT

In today's hectic environment, stress is a common occurrence in day-to-day living. Maintaining good stress management is essential for good mental and physical health. A variety of methods, such as mindfulness exercises and lifestyle modifications, are included in stress management strategies. Through the adoption of stress-reduction practices, people can lessen the detrimental effects of stress on their general health.

KNOWING THE RELATIONSHIP BETWEEN STRESS AND INFLAMMATION

Stress and inflammation are correlated in both directions. Prolonged stress can raise the body's inflammatory response, which over time may raise the chance of diseases linked to inflammation. However, inflammation can also have an impact on the brain and exacerbate symptoms associated with stress. To put successful stress management techniques into practice, it is essential to acknowledge and address this link.

RELAXATION TECHNIQUES

One of the most effective ways to combat stress and foster calmness is to incorporate relaxation techniques into your daily routine. It has been demonstrated that methods including progressive muscle relaxation, deep breathing techniques, and meditation can lower stress levels and enhance mental health in general. People might find what relaxes them the most in various scenarios by experimenting with various techniques.

OPTIMIZING YOUR SLEEP

Getting enough good sleep is essential to leading a healthy lifestyle; its significance cannot be emphasized. Immune system performance, overall cognitive function, and physical and mental recuperation all depend heavily on sleep. Making sleep a priority is essential to self-care and promotes improved general health.

IMPORTANCE OF HIGH-QUALITY SLEEP

High-quality sleep is characterized by its depth, regularity, and length. Numerous health problems have been connected to insufficient sleep, including mood swings, diminished cognitive performance, and a higher chance of developing chronic illnesses. Developing pre-sleep routines, adhering to a regular sleep schedule, and setting up a sleep-friendly atmosphere can all help you get better sleep.

ADVICE FOR DEVELOPING BETTER SLEEP HABITS

Creating a sleep-friendly atmosphere, sticking to a regular sleep schedule, and implementing pre-sleep rituals are all important steps toward developing healthy sleep habits. Practical suggestions for encouraging better sleep include minimizing screen time before bed, setting up a cozy and dark sleeping environment, and avoiding stimulants like caffeine right before bed.

CHAPTER SEVEN

SUPPLEMENTS AND PROTOCOLS FOR REDUCING INFLAMMATION

A SYNOPSIS OF SUPPLEMENTS

Supplements can help control inflammation in the body and are important for maintaining general health and well-being. For those who are interested in holistic approaches to health, it is essential to comprehend the numerous facets of supplements, such as vital nutrients, possible hazards and advantages, herbal therapies, and anti-inflammatory procedures.

CRUCIAL MINERALS FOR INFLAMMATION

An important function of essential nutrients is to control inflammation. Anti-inflammatory nutrients include antioxidants, vitamin D, and omega-3 fatty acids. It has been demonstrated that omega-3 fatty acids, which are frequently present in fish oil, can lower inflammation by preventing the synthesis of chemicals that promote inflammation. Antioxidants, which are present in fruits and vegetables, neutralize free radicals that can cause inflammation, while vitamin D, which is taken from food and sun exposure, helps to regulate the immune system.

POSSIBLE DANGERS AND ADVANTAGES

Nonetheless, it's critical to understand the advantages and possible drawbacks of using supplements. Although some supplements can have anti-inflammatory properties, overindulging in them or using them incorrectly can have negative consequences. Maintaining equilibrium and seeking advice from medical experts is essential for achieving the best possible outcomes while lowering any hazards.

HERBAL TREATMENTS

For millennia, herbal treatments have been used in many traditional healing systems. Due to their anti-inflammatory qualities, the use of herbs including Boswellia serrata, ginger, and turmeric has gained popularity. Ginger has shown promise in lowering inflammatory indicators, while turmeric, which contains curcumin, has been the subject of much research into its anti-inflammatory properties. Boswellia serrata has long been used to treat inflammatory diseases. It is made from the resin of the Boswellia tree.

CONVENTIONAL AND RESEARCH-BASED METHODS

Creating efficient anti-inflammatory regimens requires striking a balance between conventional and evidence-based methods. Combining conventional medicine with scientifically proven supplements offers a comprehensive approach to treating inflammation. Interventions supported by research provide a more sophisticated understanding of the mechanisms underlying anti-inflammatory effects, improving treatment regimens overall.

INCLUDING HERBS IN YOUR DAILY ROUTINE

Including herbs in everyday routines can be a useful strategy to make use of their anti-inflammatory properties. Consuming standardized herbal pills, brewing ginger tea, or adding turmeric to food can all help ensure regular consumption of these home cures. Individual preferences, tolerances, and possible drug interactions must all be taken into consideration.

PROTOCOLS FOR REDUCING INFLAMMATION

Anti-inflammatory regimens must be tailored to each person's requirements. The choice and dosage of supplements can be influenced by various factors, including heredity, lifestyle, and certain medical conditions. Tailored strategies provide focused interventions that target the specific variables causing inflammation in each individual.

COLLABORATING WITH MEDICAL EXPERTS

Collaboration between healthcare providers and patients is essential for anti-inflammatory measures to be successful. Healthcare professionals can evaluate each patient's current state of health, offer advice on which supplements to take, and track improvement. By incorporating expert counsel, a safe and efficient strategy is ensured, reducing potential hazards and maximizing the advantages of anti-inflammatory therapies.

Navigating the world of supplements and anti-inflammatory regimens entails appreciating the importance of key nutrients, appreciating advantages and disadvantages, investigating herbal therapies, and adopting customized strategies. Through the integration of conventional knowledge with scientifically proven methods and consulting medical experts, people can take a comprehensive approach to controlling inflammation and enhancing their general health.

CHAPTER EIGHT

MONITORING DEVELOPMENT AND MODIFYING THE PROCEDURE

KEEPING AN EYE ON INFLAMMATION LEVELS

In many medical and health situations, monitoring inflammation levels is an essential part of tracking progress and modifying regimens. One of the most important markers of the body's reaction to damage, infection, or other disruptions is inflammation. For people with long-term illnesses like autoimmune disorders or inflammatory diseases, routine measurement of inflammation levels is crucial. To track inflammation, medical professionals frequently use a mix of laboratory testing and clinical observation. This proactive strategy guarantees the best possible management of the underlying medical problem by enabling prompt modifications to treatment programs.

SCREENS AND BIOMARKERS

Tests and biomarkers are essential for accurately determining the degree of inflammation. Indicators of physiological processes that may be measured are called biomarkers, and certain biomarkers have been linked to inflammation. Pro-inflammatory cytokines, erythrocyte sedimentation rate (ESR), and C-reactive protein (CRP) are examples of common biomarkers. These indicators offer numerical information, assisting medical practitioners in impartially assessing the degree of inflammation. Furthermore, cutting-edge imaging methods like positron emission tomography (PET) and magnetic resonance imaging (MRI) provide important details on the location and intensity of inflammation in various tissues.

IDENTIFYING IMPROVEMENTS

Acknowledging improvements in a patient's state is a crucial component of the feedback loop for monitoring advancement and modifying procedures.

Positive improvements can take many different forms, depending on the illness that has to be treated. Clinical symptoms, such as less pain, increased mobility, or greater cognitive function, are closely observed by clinicians. Positive responses to therapies can also be evaluated using objective metrics, such as alterations in biomarker levels and imaging outcomes. Quality-of-life evaluations and patient-reported outcomes offer important information about how a treatment will ultimately affect a person's overall well-being.

Acknowledging beneficial changes in chronic disease goes beyond simply alleviating symptoms right away.

Remission or stabilization of the condition are examples of long-term improvements that indicate effective intervention options. To get qualitative input on patients' experiences, healthcare providers must communicate openly with their patients. By customizing protocols to meet each patient's requirements and preferences, this patient-centered approach ensures a more efficient and individualized healthcare experience.

Carefully evaluating inflammation levels, using tests and biomarkers, and identifying positive improvements come together to create a complete approach to tracking progress and making necessary protocol adjustments in healthcare.

Treatment plans can be optimized through this iterative approach, leading to better results and more patient well-being. Healthcare workers may traverse the ever-changing environment of health management with accuracy and responsiveness by adopting a comprehensive approach that integrates clinical data, patient feedback, and cutting-edge medical technologies.

MODIFYING YOUR PROCEDURE

The capacity to modify one's strategy is critical when it comes to monitoring progress and modifying protocols. Everybody's body reacts differently to different protocols, so what works for one person might not work for another. Acknowledging the necessity of adaptability in your procedure is essential to guaranteeing sustained achievement. This could include adjusting the frequency of a specific practice, changing the nutritional components, or adjusting the intensity, duration, or type of workouts in a fitness plan. Frequent self-evaluation is essential because it enables a flexible response to objectives and conditions that change. Modifying your procedure is a calculated and planned move to maximize your chances of success rather than a sign of failure.

KEEPING YOUR BODY IN MIND

A key idea in monitoring development and modifying procedures is learning to listen to your body. The body responds to different stimuli through a complex communication system. It's critical to pay attention to these indications to prevent burnout, injuries, or growth plateaus. Whether you're exercising or sticking to a diet, it's important to pay attention to small indications like weariness, discomfort, or fluctuations in energy. This self-awareness enables prompt protocol modifications, averting possible setbacks and enhancing general well-being. Ignoring these cues could result in overtraining or insufficient recovery, which would impede development and jeopardize long-term success.

LOOKING FOR EXPERT ADVICE

While having self-awareness is important, getting expert advice is just as important when it comes to monitoring development and modifying procedures. Experts in the fields of health and fitness can offer a more thorough grasp of each person's needs and the best methods. Getting advice from a fitness trainer, dietitian, or medical expert can assist in customizing protocols to meet particular needs, medical issues, and lifestyle choices. Experts can provide unbiased evaluations, tailored counsel, and evidence-based suggestions that people might not immediately recognize. This cooperative method guarantees a more comprehensive and knowledgeable approach, improving the effectiveness and long-term sustainability of advancement.

Listening to your body, changing your procedure, and getting professional advice are all interrelated and crucial steps in the process of achieving your goals and growing personally. Understanding that progress is dynamic promotes resilience, and adaptation, and keeps things from stagnating.